Doodle Reading

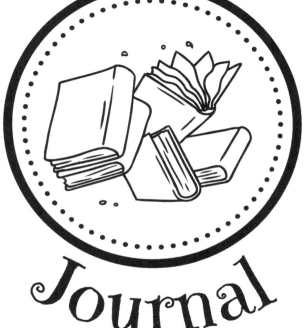

Journal

SONDERLING
PRESS

Printed by Amazon.com, Inc., in the United States of America.

First printing, 2022.

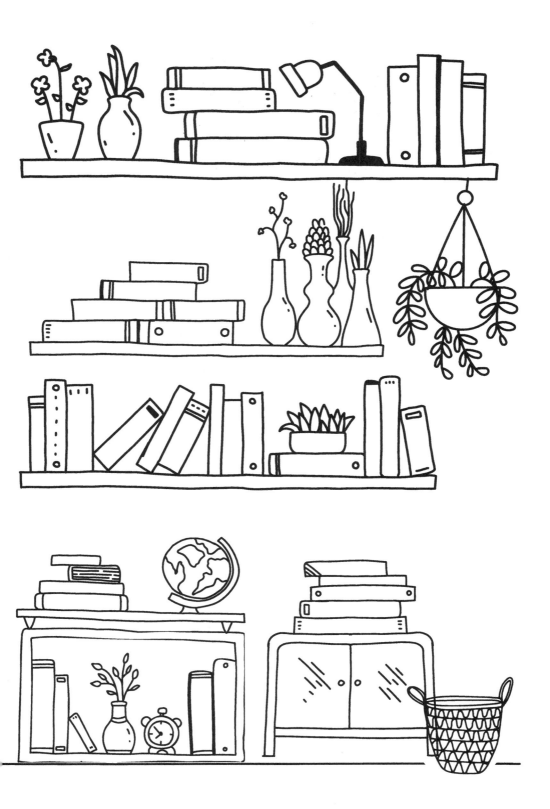

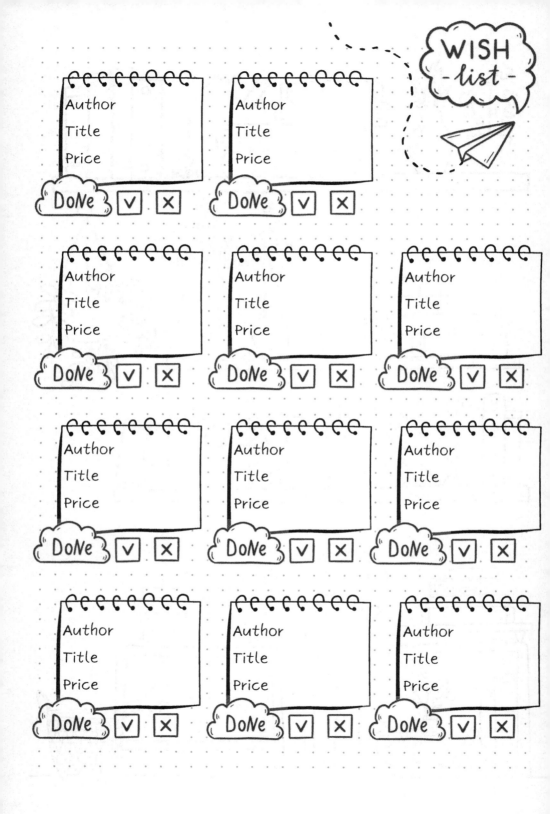

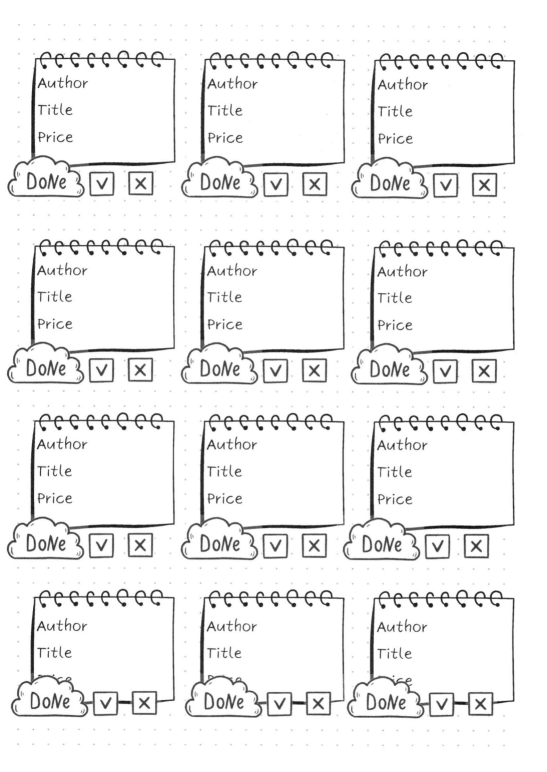

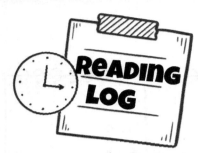

HABIT

	1	2	3	4	5	6	7	8	9	10	11	12	13	14	15
J	○	○	○	○	○	○	○	○	○	○	○	○	○	○	○
F	○	○	○	○	○	○	○	○	○	○	○	○	○	○	○
M	○	○	○	○	○	○	○	○	○	○	○	○	○	○	○
A	○	○	○	○	○	○	○	○	○	○	○	○	○	○	○
M	○	○	○	○	○	○	○	○	○	○	○	○	○	○	○
J	○	○	○	○	○	○	○	○	○	○	○	○	○	○	○
J	○	○	○	○	○	○	○	○	○	○	○	○	○	○	○
A	○	○	○	○	○	○	○	○	○	○	○	○	○	○	○
S	○	○	○	○	○	○	○	○	○	○	○	○	○	○	○
O	○	○	○	○	○	○	○	○	○	○	○	○	○	○	○
N	○	○	○	○	○	○	○	○	○	○	○	○	○	○	○
D	○	○	○	○	○	○	○	○	○	○	○	○	○	○	○

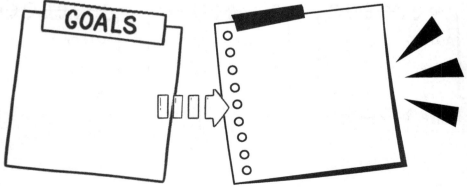

GOALS

TRACKER

16	17	18	19	20	21	22	23	24	25	26	27	28	29	30	31
○	○	○	○	○	○	○	○	○	○	○	○	○	○	○	○
○	○	○	○	○	○	○	○	○	○	○	○	○	○	○	○
○	○	○	○	○	○	○	○	○	○	○	○	○	○	○	○
○	○	○	○	○	○	○	○	○	○	○	○	○	○	○	○
○	○	○	○	○	○	○	○	○	○	○	○	○	○	○	○
○	○	○	○	○	○	○	○	○	○	○	○	○	○	○	○
○	○	○	○	○	○	○	○	○	○	○	○	○	○	○	○
○	○	○	○	○	○	○	○	○	○	○	○	○	○	○	○
○	○	○	○	○	○	○	○	○	○	○	○	○	○	○	○
○	○	○	○	○	○	○	○	○	○	○	○	○	○	○	○
○	○	○	○	○	○	○	○	○	○	○	○	○	○	○	○
○	○	○	○	○	○	○	○	○	○	○	○	○	○	○	○

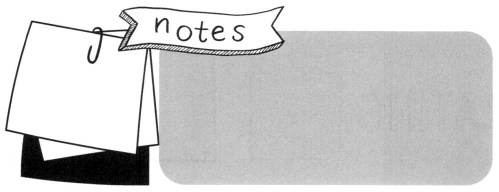

notes

Book Review

Recommend?

☑ ☒

To who

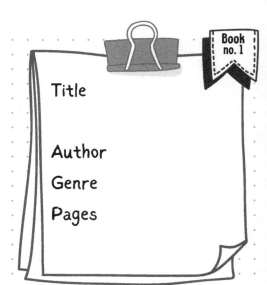

Book no. 1

Title

Author
Genre
Pages

summary

Start Date
....
Finish Date
....

favourite QUOTE

RATING

☆ ☆ ☆ ☆ ☆

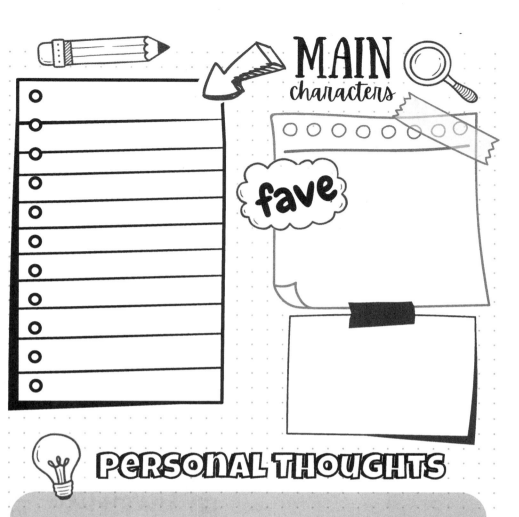

MAIN characters

fave

PERSONAL THOUGHTS

Book Review

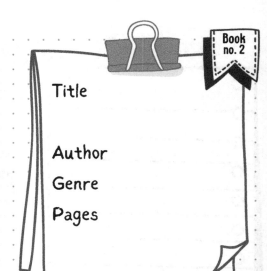

Book no. 2

Title

Author

Genre

Pages

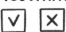

Recommend?

☑ ☒

To who

summary

Start Date
....

Finish Date
....

♥ favourite QUOTE

RATING

☆ ☆ ☆ ☆ ☆

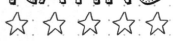

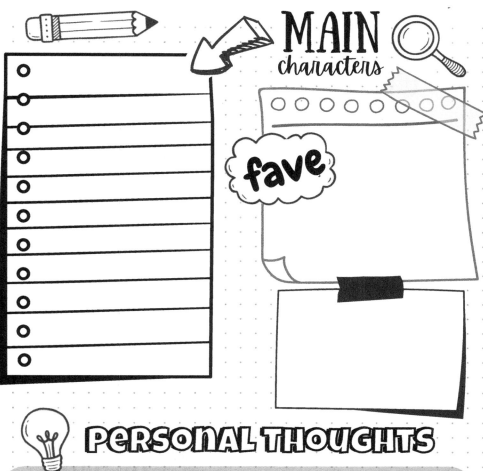

MAIN characters

fave

PERSONAL THOUGHTS

Book Review

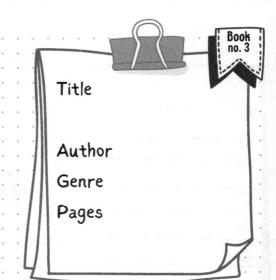

Book no. 3

Title

Author

Genre

Pages

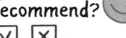

Recommend?

☑ ☒

To who

Summary

Start Date
....
Finish Date
....

Favourite QUOTE

RATING

☆ ☆ ☆ ☆ ☆

MAIN characters

fave

PERSONAL THOUGHTS

Book Review

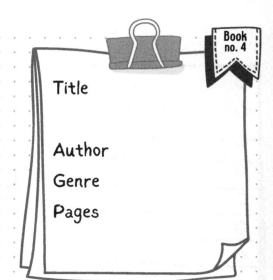

Book no. 4

Title

Author

Genre

Pages

Recommend?

☑ ☒

To who

Summary

Start Date

....

Finish Date

....

Favourite QUOTE

RATING

☆ ☆ ☆ ☆ ☆

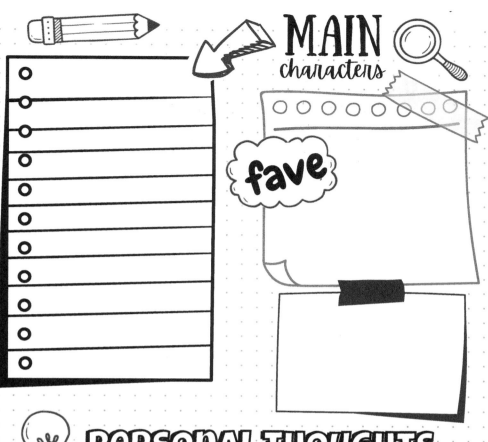

MAIN characters

fave

PERSONAL THOUGHTS

Book Review

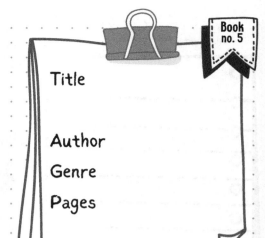

Book no. 5

Title

Author

Genre

Pages

Recommend?

☑ ☒

To who

Summary

Start Date
....

Finish Date
....

Favourite QUOTE

RATING

☆ ☆ ☆ ☆ ☆

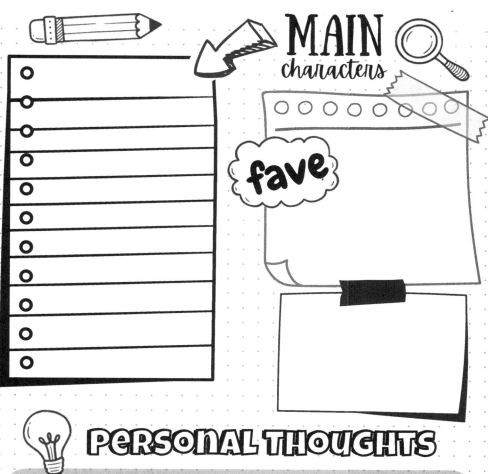

MAIN characters

fave

PERSONAL THOUGHTS

Book Review

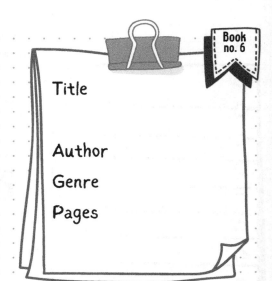

Book no. 6

Title

Author

Genre

Pages

Recommend? 🙂

☑ ☒

To who

summary

Start Date

....

Finish Date

....

Favourite QUOTE

RATING

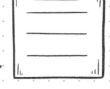

☆ ☆ ☆ ☆ ☆

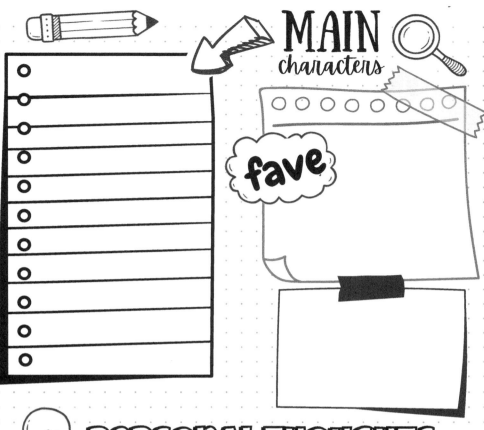

MAIN characters

fave

PERSONAL THOUGHTS

Book Review

Recommend?
☑ ☒
To who

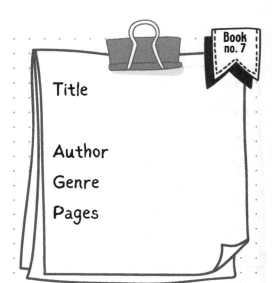

Book no. 7

Title

Author

Genre

Pages

summary

Start Date
....
Finish Date
....

♥ Favourite QUOTE

RATING
☆ ☆ ☆ ☆ ☆

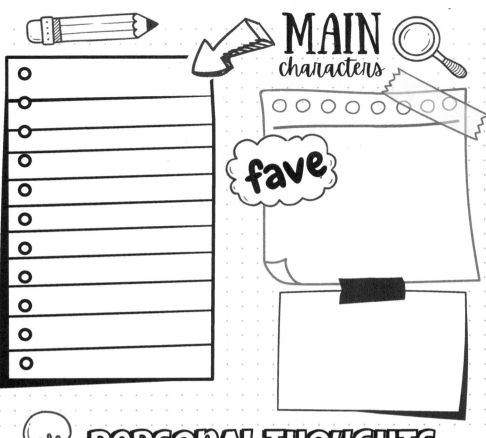

MAIN characters

fave

PERSONAL THOUGHTS

Book Review

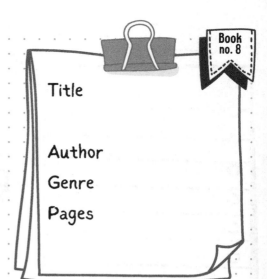

Book no. 8

Title

Author

Genre

Pages

Recommend?

☑ ☒

To who

summary

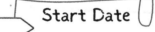

Start Date ....

Finish Date ....

favourite QUOTE

RATING

☆ ☆ ☆ ☆ ☆

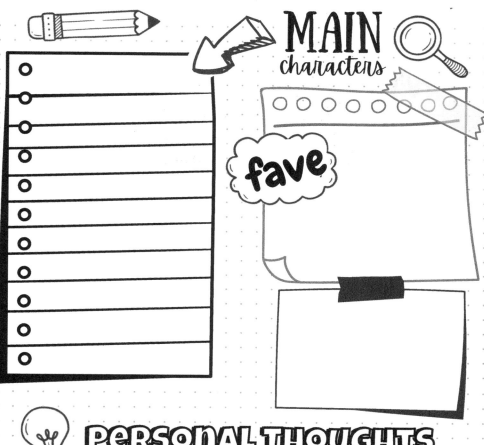

MAIN characters

fave

 PERSONAL THOUGHTS

Book Review

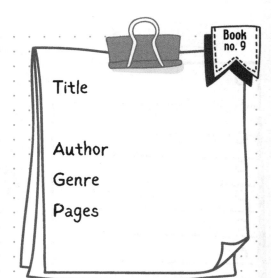

Book no. 9

Title

Author

Genre

Pages

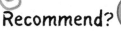

Recommend? ☺

☑ ☒

To who

summary

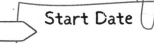

Start Date

·····················

Finish Date

·····················

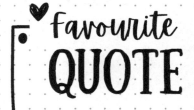

♥ Favourite QUOTE

RATING

☆ ☆ ☆ ☆ ☆

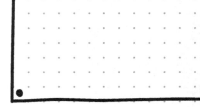

MAIN characters

fave

PERSONAL THOUGHTS

Book Review

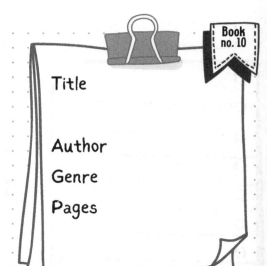

Book no. 10

Title

Author
Genre
Pages

Recommend?

To who

summary

Start Date
....
Finish Date
....

favourite QUOTE

RATING

☆ ☆ ☆ ☆ ☆

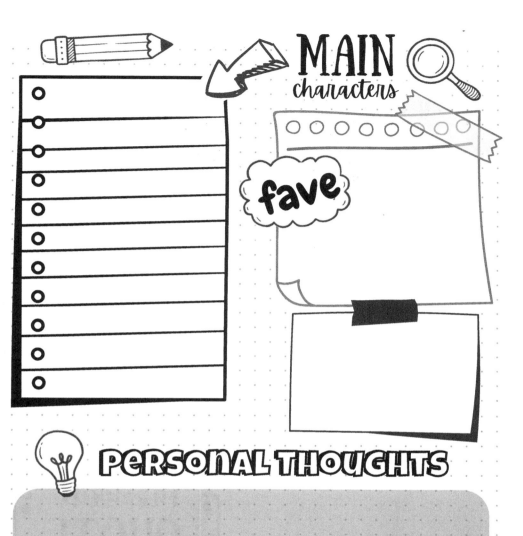

MAIN characters

fave

PERSONAL THOUGHTS

Book Review

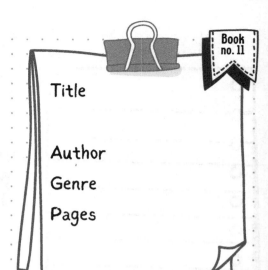

Book no. 11

Title

Author
Genre
Pages

Recommend?

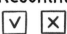

☑   ☒

To who

Summary

Start Date
....

Finish Date
....

Favourite QUOTE

RATING

☆ ☆ ☆ ☆ ☆

MAIN characters

fave

PERSONAL THOUGHTS

Book Review

Recommend?

To who

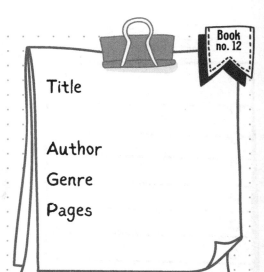

Book no. 12

Title

Author

Genre

Pages

Summary

Start Date
....
Finish Date
....

Favourite QUOTE

RATING

☆ ☆ ☆ ☆ ☆

MAIN characters

fave

PERSONAL THOUGHTS

Book Review

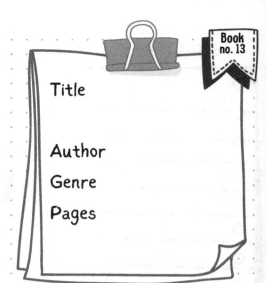

Book no. 13

Title

Author

Genre

Pages

Recommend?

☑ ☒

To who

summary

Start Date
....
Finish Date
....

Favourite QUOTE

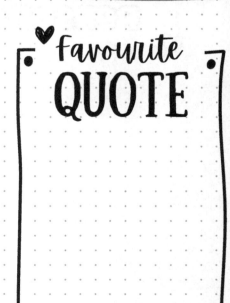

RATING

☆ ☆ ☆ ☆ ☆

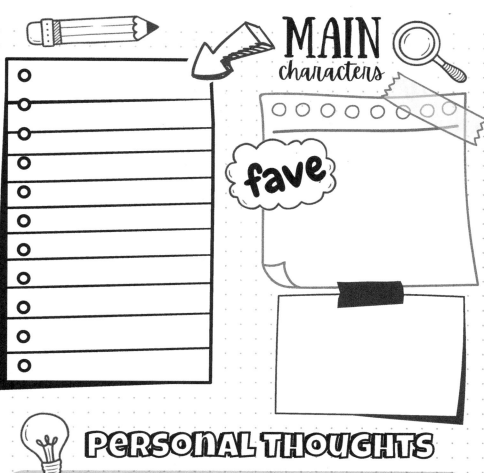

MAIN characters

fave

PERSONAL THOUGHTS

Book Review

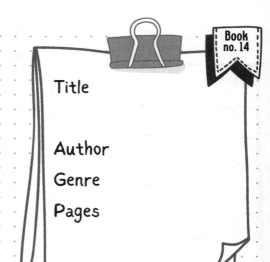

Book no. 14

Title

Author

Genre

Pages

Recommend?

☑ ☒

To who

summary

Start Date

....

Finish Date

....

Favourite QUOTE

RATING

☆ ☆ ☆ ☆ ☆

MAIN characters

fave

PERSONAL THOUGHTS

Book Review

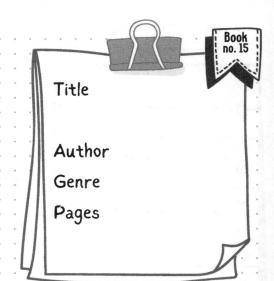

Book no. 15

Title

Author
Genre
Pages

Recommend?

[✓] [✗]

To who

summary

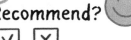

Start Date
....
Finish Date
....

Favourite QUOTE

RATING

☆ ☆ ☆ ☆ ☆

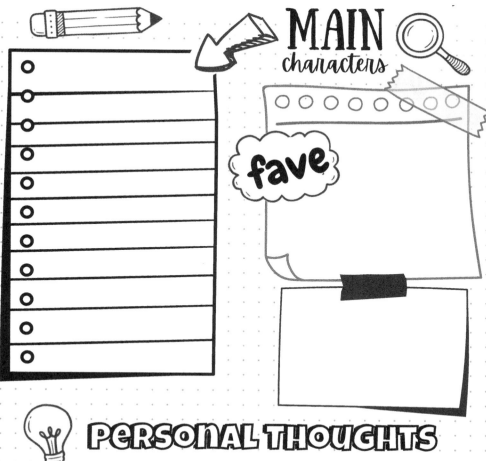

MAIN characters

fave

PERSONAL THOUGHTS

Book Review

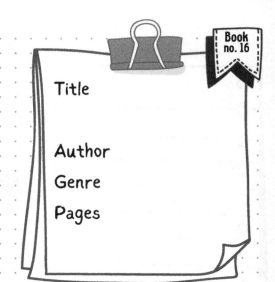

Book no. 16

Title

Author

Genre

Pages

Recommend?

☑ ☒

To who

Summary

Start Date

....

Finish Date

....

♥ Favourite QUOTE

RATING

☆ ☆ ☆ ☆ ☆

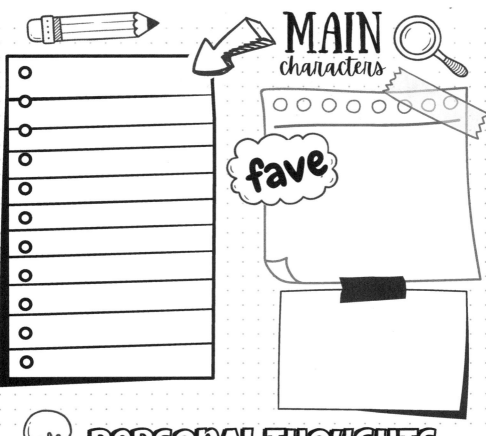

MAIN characters

fave

PERSONAL THOUGHTS

Book Review

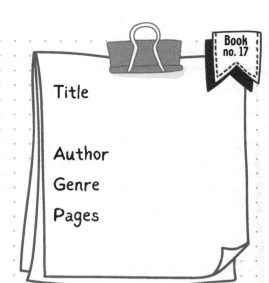

Book no. 17

Title

Author

Genre

Pages

Recommend?

[✓] [✗]

To who

summary

Start Date

....

Finish Date

....

♥ Favourite

QUOTE

RATING

☆ ☆ ☆ ☆ ☆

MAIN characters

fave

PERSONAL THOUGHTS

Book Review

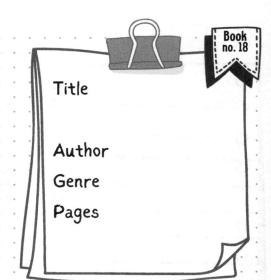

Book no. 18

Title

Author

Genre

Pages

Recommend?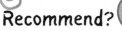

☑ ☒

To who

summary

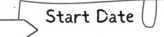

Start Date

Finish Date

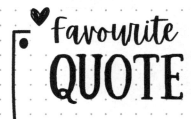

Favourite QUOTE

RATING

☆ ☆ ☆ ☆ ☆

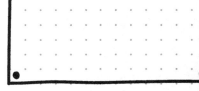

MAIN characters

fave

PERSONAL THOUGHTS

Book Review

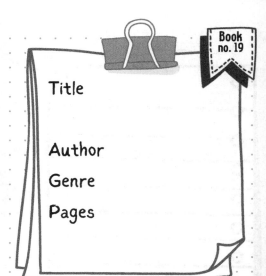

Book no. 19

Title

Author

Genre

Pages

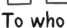

Recommend? ☺

☑ ☒

To who

summary

Start Date

....

Finish Date

....

♥ Favourite QUOTE

RATING

☆ ☆ ☆ ☆ ☆

MAIN characters

fave

PERSONAL THOUGHTS

Book Review

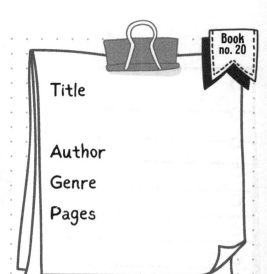

Book no. 20

Title

Author
Genre
Pages

Recommend? 🙂

☑ ☒

To who

summary

Start Date
....

Finish Date
....

♥ favourite QUOTE

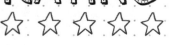 RATING

☆ ☆ ☆ ☆ ☆

MAIN characters

fave

PERSONAL THOUGHTS

Book Review

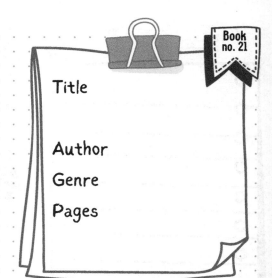

Book no. 21

Title

Author

Genre

Pages

Recommend?

[✓] [✗]

To who

summary

Start Date
....

Finish Date
....

Favourite QUOTE

RATING

☆ ☆ ☆ ☆ ☆

MAIN characters

fave

PERSONAL THOUGHTS

Book Review

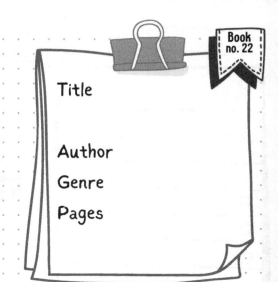

Book no. 22

Title

Author

Genre

Pages

Recommend?

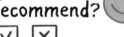

☑ ☒

To who

summary

Start Date

....

Finish Date

....

Favourite QUOTE

RATING

☆ ☆ ☆ ☆ ☆

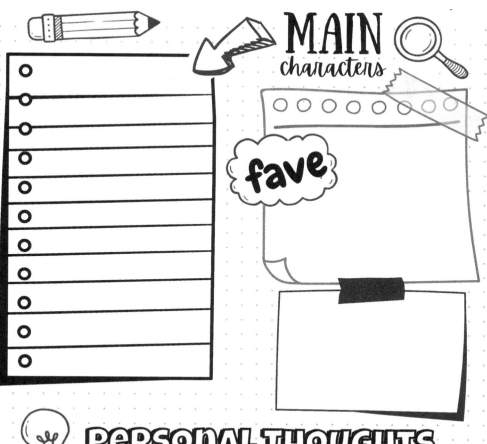

MAIN characters

fave

PERSONAL THOUGHTS

Book Review

Recommend? 🙂
☑ ☒
To who

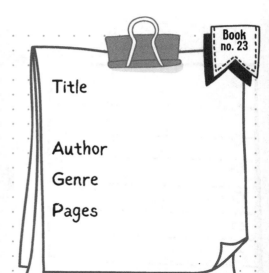

Book no. 23

Title

Author
Genre
Pages

summary

Start Date
....
Finish Date
....

♥ Favourite
QUOTE

RATING
☆ ☆ ☆ ☆ ☆

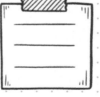

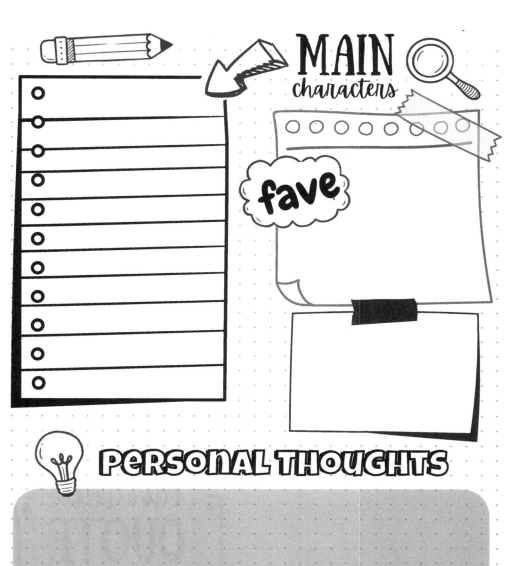

MAIN characters

fave

PERSONAL THOUGHTS

Book Review

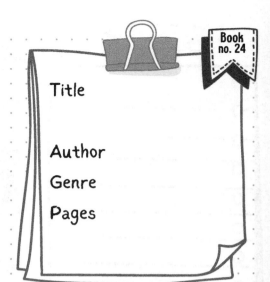

Book no. 24

Title

Author

Genre

Pages

Recommend?

[✓] [✗]

To who

summary

Start Date
....
Finish Date
....

Favourite QUOTE

RATING

☆ ☆ ☆ ☆ ☆

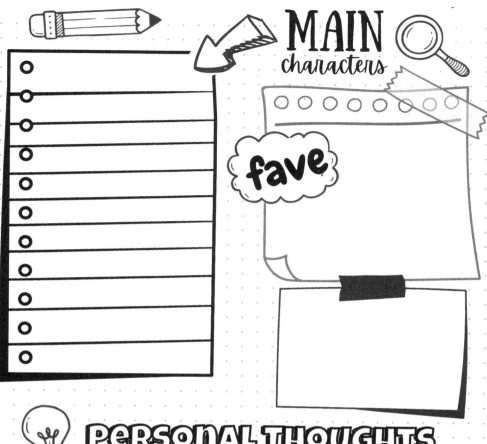

MAIN characters

fave

PERSONAL THOUGHTS

Book Review

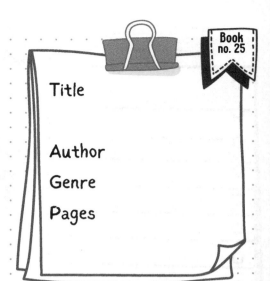

Book no. 25

Title

Author

Genre

Pages

Recommend? 🙂

☑ ☒

To who

summary

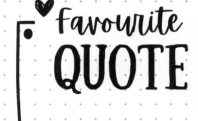

Start Date

....

Finish Date

....

♡ Favourite QUOTE

RATING

☆ ☆ ☆ ☆ ☆

MAIN characters

fave

PERSONAL THOUGHTS

Book Review

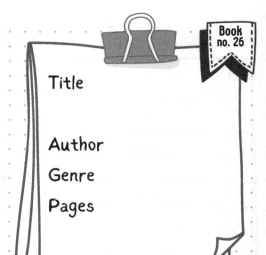

Book no. 26

Title

Author
Genre
Pages

Recommend? 🙂
☑ ☒
To who

summary

Start Date
....
Finish Date
....

Favourite QUOTE

RATING
☆ ☆ ☆ ☆ ☆

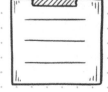

MAIN characters

fave

PERSONAL THOUGHTS

Book Review

Recommend?
☑ ☒
To who

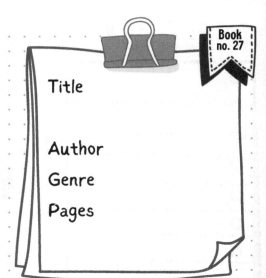

Book no. 27

Title

Author
Genre
Pages

summary

Start Date
....
Finish Date
....

♥ Favourite
QUOTE

RATING

☆ ☆ ☆ ☆ ☆

MAIN characters

fave

PERSONAL THOUGHTS

Book Review

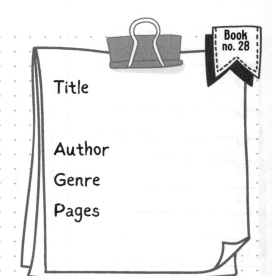

Book no. 28

Title

Author

Genre

Pages

Recommend?

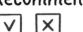

☑ ☒

To who

summary

Start Date
....
Finish Date
....

favourite QUOTE

RATING

☆ ☆ ☆ ☆ ☆

MAIN characters

fave

PERSONAL THOUGHTS

Book Review

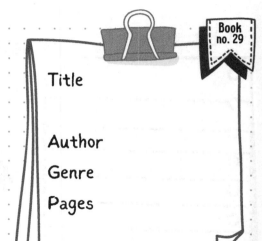

Book no. 29

Title

Author

Genre

Pages

Recommend?

☑ ☒

To who

summary

Start Date

....

Finish Date

....

favourite QUOTE

RATING

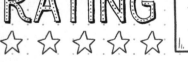

☆ ☆ ☆ ☆ ☆

MAIN characters

fave

PERSONAL THOUGHTS

Book Review

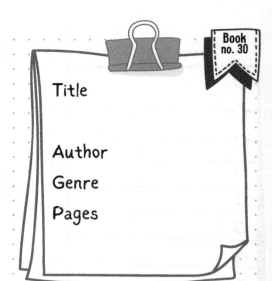

Book no. 30

Title

Author

Genre

Pages

Recommend?
☑ ☒
To who

summary

Start Date

Finish Date

Favourite QUOTE

RATING

☆ ☆ ☆ ☆ ☆

MAIN characters

fave

PERSONAL THOUGHTS

Book Review

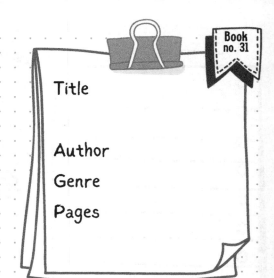

Book no. 31

Title

Author

Genre

Pages

Recommend?

☑ ☒

To who

summary

Start Date

....

Finish Date

....

Favourite QUOTE

RATING

☆ ☆ ☆ ☆ ☆

MAIN characters

fave

PERSONAL THOUGHTS

Book Review

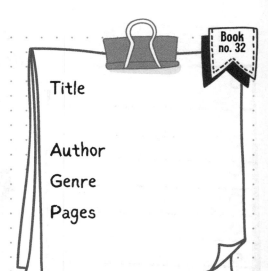

Book no. 32

Title

Author

Genre

Pages

Recommend?

☑ ☒

To who

summary

Start Date

....

Finish Date

....

♥ Favourite QUOTE

RATING

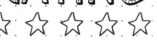

⭐ ⭐ ⭐ ⭐ ⭐

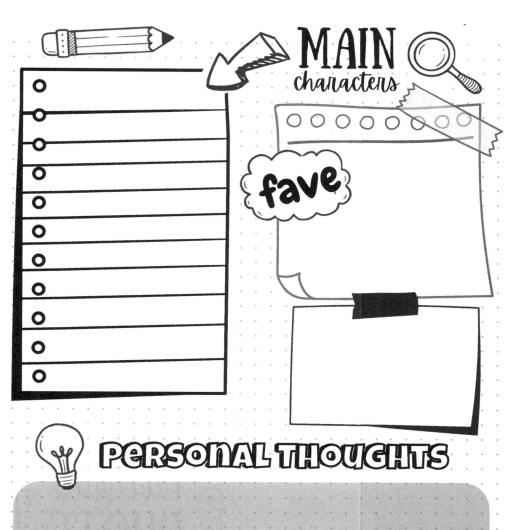

MAIN characters

fave

PERSONAL THOUGHTS

Book Review

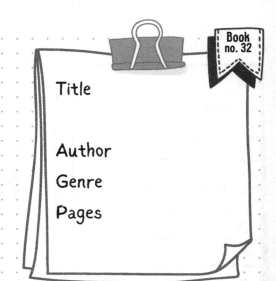

Book no. 32

Title

Author

Genre

Pages

Recommend?

☑ ☒

To who

summary

Start Date
....

Finish Date
....

Favourite QUOTE

RATING

☆ ☆ ☆ ☆ ☆

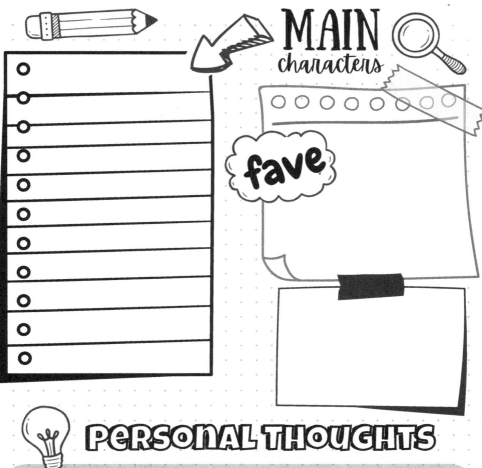

MAIN characters

fave

PERSONAL THOUGHTS

Book Review

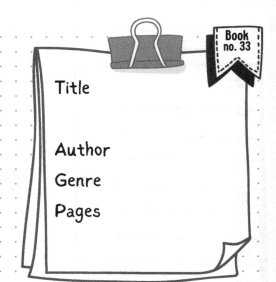

Book no. 33

Title

Author

Genre

Pages

Recommend?

☑ ☒

To who

summary

Start Date

....

Finish Date

....

Favourite QUOTE

RATING

☆ ☆ ☆ ☆ ☆

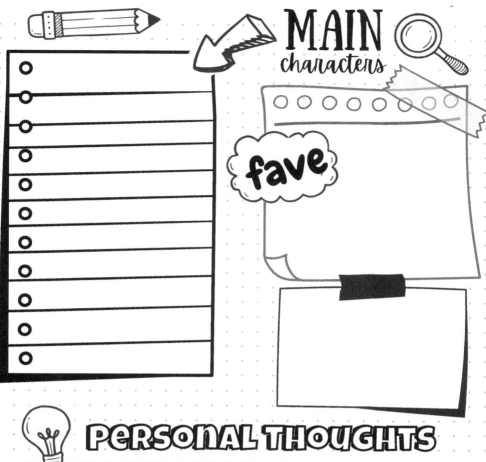

MAIN characters

fave

PERSONAL THOUGHTS

Book Review

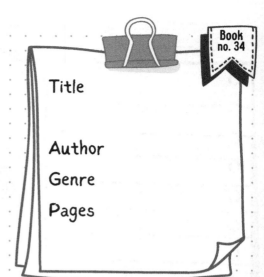

Book no. 34

Title

Author

Genre

Pages

Recommend?

☑ ☒

To who

summary

Start Date

Finish Date

favourite QUOTE

RATING

☆ ☆ ☆ ☆ ☆

MAIN characters

fave

PERSONAL THOUGHTS

Book Review

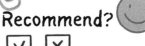

Recommend? :)

[✓] [✗]

To who

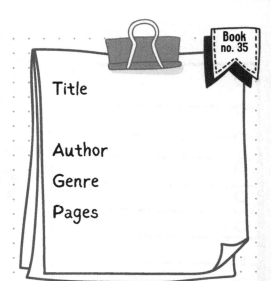

Book no. 35

Title

Author

Genre

Pages

summary

Start Date
....
Finish Date
....

♡ Favourite QUOTE

RATING

☆ ☆ ☆ ☆ ☆

MAIN characters

fave

PERSONAL THOUGHTS

Book Review

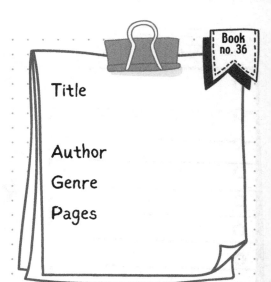

Book no. 36

Title

Author

Genre

Pages

Recommend?

☑ ☒

To who

Summary

Start Date

Finish Date

Favourite QUOTE

RATING

☆ ☆ ☆ ☆ ☆

MAIN characters

fave

PERSONAL THOUGHTS

Book Review

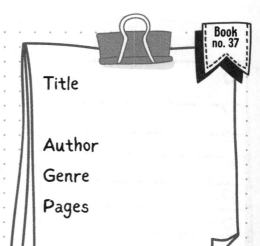

Book no. 37

Title

Author
Genre
Pages

Recommend?
[✓] [✗]
To who

summary

Start Date
....
Finish Date
....

Favourite QUOTE

RATING
☆ ☆ ☆ ☆ ☆

MAIN
characters

fave

PERSONAL THOUGHTS

Book Review

Recommend?
[✓] [✗]
To who

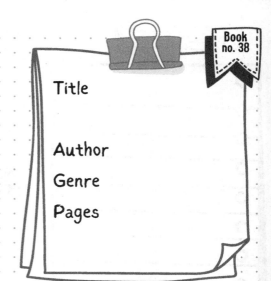

Book no. 38

Title

Author
Genre
Pages

summary

Start Date
....
Finish Date
....

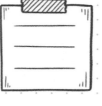

Favourite QUOTE

RATING
☆ ☆ ☆ ☆ ☆

MAIN
characters

fave

PERSONAL THOUGHTS

Book Review

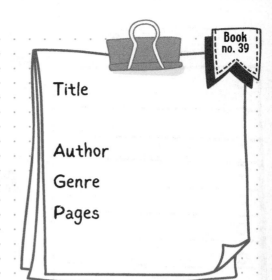

Book no. 39

Title

Author

Genre

Pages

Recommend?

☑ ☒

To who

summary

Start Date
....
Finish Date
....

favourite QUOTE

RATING

☆ ☆ ☆ ☆ ☆

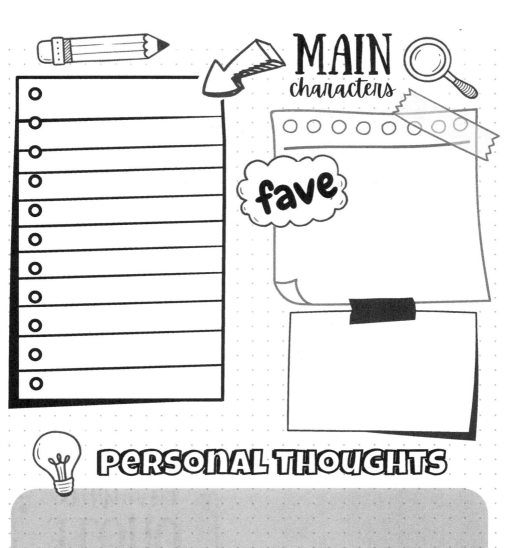

MAIN characters

fave

PERSONAL THOUGHTS

Book Review

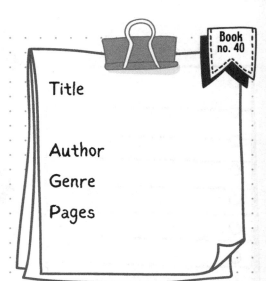

Book no. 40

Title

Author

Genre

Pages

Recommend?

☑ ☒

To who

Summary

Start Date
....
Finish Date
....

Favourite QUOTE

RATING

☆ ☆ ☆ ☆ ☆

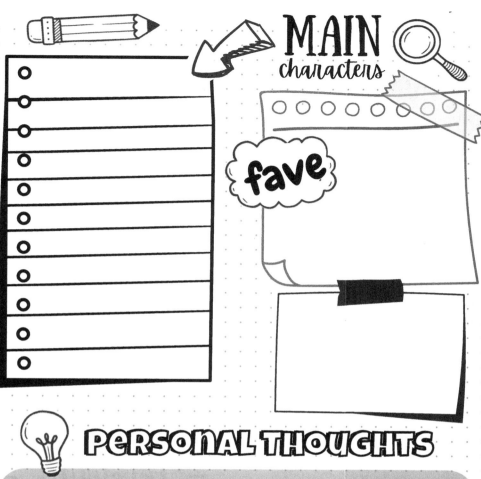

MAIN
characters

fave

PERSONAL THOUGHTS

Book Review

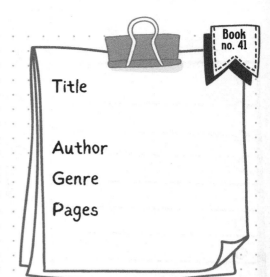

Book no. 41

Title

Author

Genre

Pages

Recommend?

☑ ☒

To who

Summary

Start Date

....

Finish Date

....

Favourite QUOTE

RATING

☆ ☆ ☆ ☆ ☆

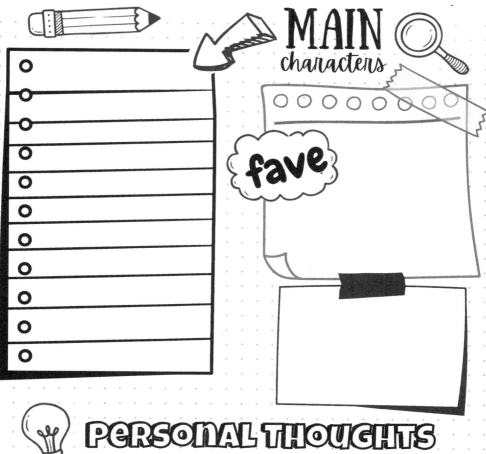

MAIN characters

fave

PERSONAL THOUGHTS

Book Review

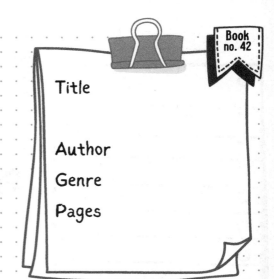

Book no. 42

Title

Author

Genre

Pages

Recommend?

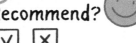

☑ ☒

To who

summary

Start Date

....

Finish Date

....

♥ favourite QUOTE

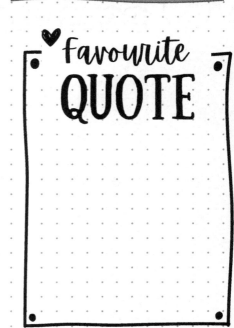

RATING

☆ ☆ ☆ ☆ ☆

MAIN characters

fave

PERSONAL THOUGHTS

Book Review

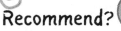

Recommend?
☑ ☒
To who

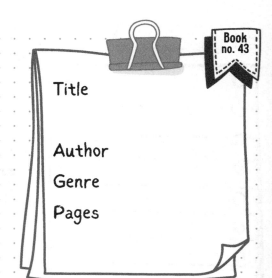

Book no. 43

Title

Author

Genre

Pages

summary

Start Date
....
Finish Date
....

Favourite QUOTE

RATING

☆ ☆ ☆ ☆ ☆

MAIN characters

fave

PERSONAL THOUGHTS

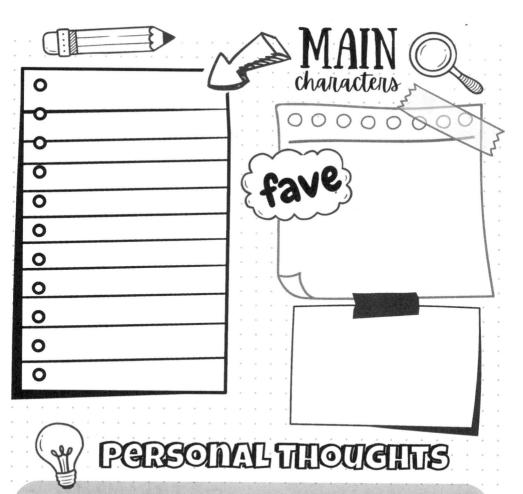

Book Review

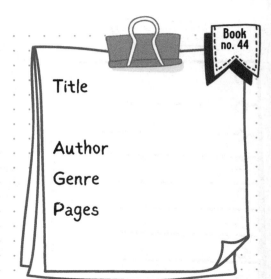

Book no. 44

Title

Author

Genre

Pages

Recommend?

☑ ☒

To who

summary

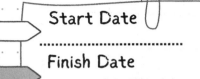

Start Date

....

Finish Date

....

Favourite QUOTE

RATING

☆ ☆ ☆ ☆ ☆

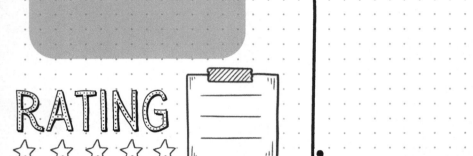

MAIN characters

fave

PERSONAL THOUGHTS

Book Review

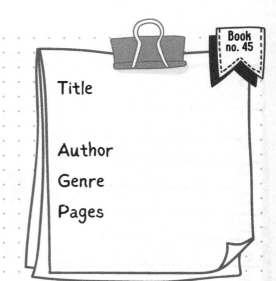

Book no. 45

Title

Author

Genre

Pages

Recommend?

☑ ☒

To who

summary

Start Date
....
Finish Date
....

favourite QUOTE

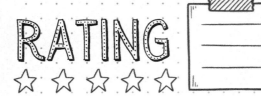

RATING

☆ ☆ ☆ ☆ ☆

MAIN characters

fave

PERSONAL THOUGHTS

Book Review

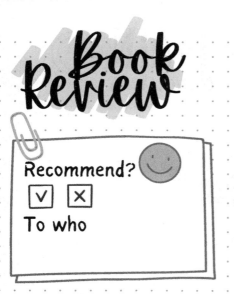

Recommend?
[✓] [✗]
To who

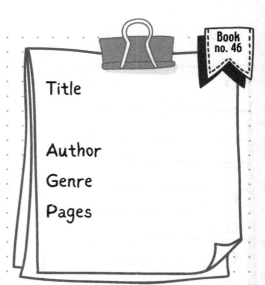

Book no. 46

Title

Author
Genre
Pages

Summary

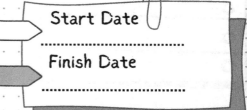

Start Date
....
Finish Date
....

Favourite QUOTE

RATING

☆ ☆ ☆ ☆ ☆

MAIN characters

fave

PERSONAL THOUGHTS

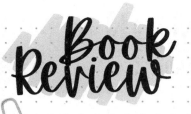

Book Review

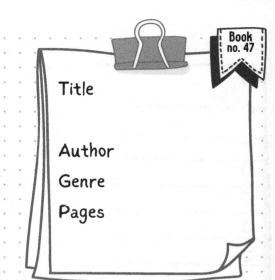

Book no. 47

Title

Author
Genre
Pages

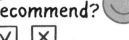

Recommend?

☑ ☒

To who

Summary

Start Date
....
Finish Date
....

Favourite QUOTE

RATING

☆ ☆ ☆ ☆ ☆

MAIN
characters

fave

PERSONAL THOUGHTS

Book Review

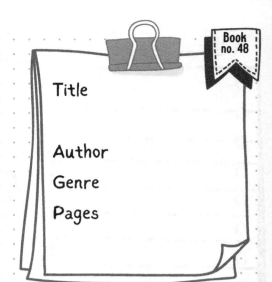

Book no. 48

Title

Author

Genre

Pages

Recommend?

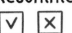

☑ ☒

To who

summary

Start Date
....

Finish Date
....

Favourite QUOTE

RATING

☆ ☆ ☆ ☆ ☆

MAIN characters

fave

PERSONAL THOUGHTS

Book Review

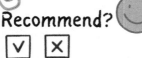

Recommend? 🙂

[✓] [✗]

To who

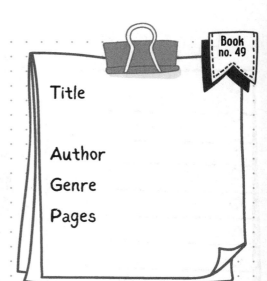

Book no. 49

Title

Author

Genre

Pages

summary

Start Date
....

Finish Date
....

Favourite QUOTE

RATING

☆ ☆ ☆ ☆ ☆

MAIN characters

fave

PERSONAL THOUGHTS

Book Review

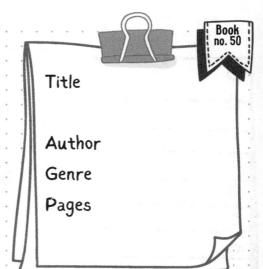

Book no. 50

Title

Author
Genre
Pages

Recommend?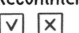

☑ ☒
To who

summary

Start Date
....
Finish Date
....

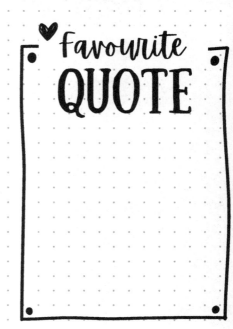

Favourite QUOTE

RATING

☆ ☆ ☆ ☆ ☆

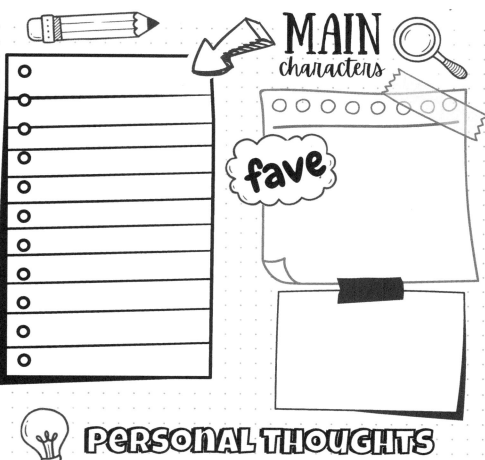

MAIN characters

fave

PERSONAL THOUGHTS

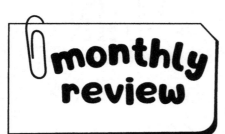 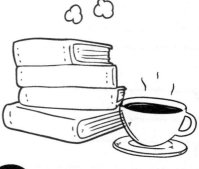

monthly review

1

How many books I read:

My favorite book:

Least favorite book:

4

How many books I read:

My favorite book:

Least favorite book:

2

How many books I read:

My favorite book:

Least favorite book:

5

How many books I read:

My favorite book:

Least favorite book:

3

How many books I read:

My favorite book:

Least favorite book:

6

How many books I read:

My favorite book:

Least favorite book:

7 How many books I read:

My favorite book:

Least favorite book:

10 How many books I read:

My favorite book:

Least favorite book:

8 How many books I read:

My favorite book:

Least favorite book:

11 How many books I read:

My favorite book:

Least favorite book:

9 How many books I read:

My favorite book:

Least favorite book:

12 How many books I read:

My favorite book:

Least favorite book:

LIBRARY
BOOK TRACKER

Title	Borrow Date	Return Date

Title	Borrow Date	Return Date

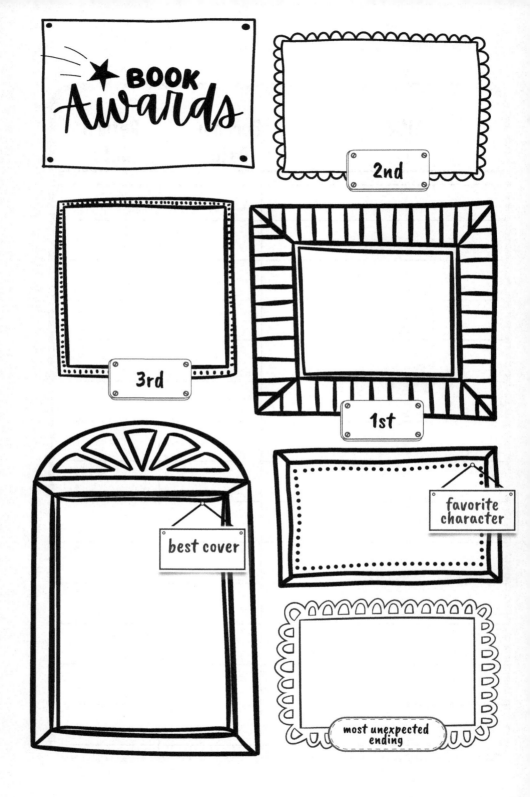

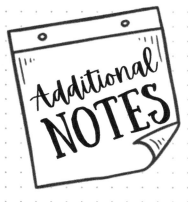

Made in the USA
Middletown, DE
14 October 2023